Ordering Information:

Quantity sales. Special discounts are available on quantity purchases
by corporations, associations, and others. Orders by U.S. trade
bookstores and wholesalers.

Printed in the United States of America

First Printing, 2016

ISBN-13: 978-1539331568

ISBN-10: 1539331563

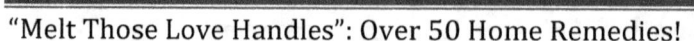

Disclaimer (My Lawyer Made Me Write This):

"Any exercise is not without inherent risks and any exercises may result in injury or illness. We therefore advise you to consult a doctor before attempting any physical exercise program."

Table of Contents:

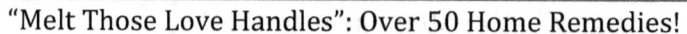

Learning to Love Your Body

"Your body is precious. It is our vehicle for awakening. Treat it with care." ~Buddha

Let's start off this journey together. I am here for you. I originally did not start out by writing this book. This is a collection of my blog posts I have been writing for the last 5 years. But I have had so much positive feedback from my wonderful followers, I wanted to turn it into a book.

The purpose of this book is to educate you on the healthy food choices you can make which will reduce your love handles. But first, before we begin on the physical body, let's take time to focus on our spiritual and emotional selves. There is a direct connection from your inner world to your outer world. I truly believe that the way we feel on the outside (the body we see in the mirror) is directly related from the way we feel on the inside (our self-image of ourselves). The following pages leading up to the actual food choices were purposely included in this book (despite my publisher's advice!) because these mindsets have helped me to achieve my perfect body and a healthy soul. If you practice these mindsets I trust they will help you too.

In order for you to trust me, let me give you the story of my life. As long as I can remember, I've always hated my body. I hated the way it looked in the mirror. The oval shape, the love handles which seems to extend off of my body. My life has been one big hate fest of my body. For as long as I can remember, I always hated my physical self. I don't know when or how it developed, but I have been comparing my body to others' for as long as I can remember. I was never happy, never good enough. There was always work to be done, goals to achieve, people to impress. I always covered up at the beach. Just the thought of wearing a bathing suit was enough start my anxiety. Of course, I never reached any of my goals.

Not only was I constantly on the latest fade diet that most likely was extremely bad for me, but I was also mentally beating myself up every step of the way. Why was I doing this to myself? The self-talk was brutal and relentless. "Why are my love handles so big! "Why can't I just lose weight?" "Why am I so fat?" The negativity didn't stop there. I hated others too. Women and men with "perfect" bodies were a major source of jealousy and envy for me. God, I hated my love handles.

The few times that I achieved some sort of ideal, I found myself uncomfortable with my appearance. I guess call it fate, but I projected my hatred and jealousy of others onto myself, and just kept falling down the negativity rabbit hole. Minor achievements felt shallow, undeserved, and were always short-lived and followed by a period of self-sabotage.

Finally, after a difficult separation and divorce, left as a single mother raising two young children alone, some sort of light bulb went off in my head. I am in my late 30's and no one else was going to take care of me. I was sick of the misery and mental anguish. I realized more than ever that I needed to take care of myself so that I could have the energy to get through my demanding life. Something had to give, and what I was doing was not working. I began by simply realizing that I didn't feel good physically with the way that I was eating. I noticed a daily sugar crash that was leaving me depressed and with no energy. I was totally depleted after work. I was missing out on spending happy times with my children. I decided to start there and started eating more whole foods and less sugar.

I soon realized something and it totally changed my life. Taking a new attitude toward my diet increased my awareness of how good health affected me, and that choice built upon itself daily. I researched what else I could do to develop better health, and began to properly care for myself. In turn, my life became more manageable, I felt happier, and I was a better mom and person. As a nice bonus I actually lost 35 pounds and became an avid runner. My love handles disappeared!

If you're tired of the self-hate game and ready to begin taking care of yourself, you may want to try the steps that I followed.

Focus on feeling well.

Stop obsessing over external appearances and obtaining an ideal body, like the ones you see on those magazine covers, and instead focus on the way being healthy makes you feel and what it gives you. You see, there is no "ideal body". You'll find a deeper sense of gratification and more motivation to stay on track. You'll also begin to lose tolerance for the way unhealthy choices make you feel. Besides, those people you see on those covers are paid models and do not look like that on a Dailey basis.

You can also reframe the way you look at diet and exercise as something wonderful you do for yourself, rather than a way to punish your unhealthy choices. Don't look at it as a chore, but as a way to nurture yourself. Feed your body nourishing food so that you always feel your best, and remove the worries of disease and poor health. Exercise to relieve the daily stresses of life, to release endorphins, to fight anxiety, and to feel good. Do it for yourself! Meditate to get in touch with your emotions, to connect with the bigger picture, and to feel at peace.

The Golden Rule

Treat yourself the way you'd treat someone you love. I stopped speaking to myself in a way that I wouldn't speak to my children or an adult. It's powerful to recognize that the self-hatred is not only unproductive, but that it begins a spiral that takes you further and further away from the things that you want. How motivated would you feel to perform well for a boss who constantly demeaned you? Now imagine a boss who supported, encouraged, and nurtured you: how motivated would you be then?

Our subconscious mind hears the self-talk and responds to it in a similar way, so make sure your self-talk is loving, supportive, nurturing, and forgiving. Look in the mirror every day and repeat the phrase "I am deserving and worthy of all good things, and accept myself unconditionally." I am a fan of Louise Hay's work. Practicing her affirmations on a consistent basis has changed my life. You should YouTube her videos and listen to them. They will change your life as it did mine.

It may take some time to believe it, but in time you will re-train your thought process to be more positive. When a negative thought about yourself enters your head, take a deep breath, release it, and repeat your positive affirmation in its place. If you're not sure, ask yourself "Would I say this to my daughter/son/loved one?" Treat yourself with the utmost respect, and you will want to give your body the healthy choices that it deserves and needs to function in the best way possible.

Stay positive and be grateful.

Don't waste time and emotions staring at pictures of perfect bodies and wishing to be one of them. If you need visual inspiration, find photos of *you* at *your* best, not someone else at *their* best. Learn to release negative thoughts about your body and to focus on the good that it brings you every single day. Rather than fixating on not having lost that five pounds yet, or not fitting into that dress yet, make a daily list of your accomplishments and your gratitude.

Just like in the rest of life, when we focus on what we don't have or what we haven't accomplished, we feel frustrated and ready to give up. Listing your achievements instead puts your focus on what is going right, which in turn motivates you to do more.

Realize, that the best you can do is not all you can do. Maybe when you started, you couldn't do one single push-up—and now you can do 10. That's huge! No accomplishment is too small to be grateful for, because it has taken you one more step in the right direction. There is now no reason to give up, because with this attitude, you cannot fail.

Love yourself first

Love yourself first and the rest will follow. Learn to love yourself by catching and releasing negative thoughts, acknowledging your efforts and achievements, making positive daily affirmations, and seeing perfection in your so-called "imperfections." Ironically enough, focusing on loving and caring for yourself first will most likely lead to the external transformation that you've always wanted. Once you begin to treat yourself with the respect and care that you deserve, the habits needed for physical transformation develop naturally.

You'll want to nourish your body because you are grateful for it, so healthy choices will come with ease. When an unhealthy choice makes you feel awful, you won't stand for it because you know you deserve better. Before you know it, you'll see your body transform, and not just in fat/muscle composition, but a healthy glow from the inside out.I can now look in the mirror, smile, and be happy with what I see, no matter *what* I see. Part of my beauty is the light that shines from within. I am at peace with myself.

Self-Image

Self- Image is the most important concept I ever learned and I want to share it with you. This concept has what kept the weight down and love handles off. In this section you will learn that the reason you fail to achieve your goals is probably your self-image, you will never be able to maintain better results than your self-image, and in order to change it, you must use autosuggestion.

Modern psychology shows us that 95% of our actions are habitual. This means that 95% of what we do happens without conscious thought. **What really controls our behavior is the image we have of ourselves in our mind. That image is the pattern by which we live our lives.**

I learned this from "You were Born Rich" by Bob Proctor – one of the leading authors and speakers on human potential. At one point in the book Bob says something I shall never forget: *"The part of you that knows is not the part that controls your behavior. Long term habit change is NEVER the result of a strong willpower. Long term results are always, ALWAYS equal to your self-image."*

Let's repeat that:

"Long term results are always, ALWAYS equal to your self-image."

Have you noticed that? Have you noticed that your life is exactly the way you picture it in your mind?

You have as much money as you see yourself having. You have the type of clothes you see yourself wearing. Your body always looks like the way you see it in your mind. Your home looks the way you picture it in your mind. And of course, you have the type of success you see yourself having.

Maxwell Maltz was the doctor who popularized the study of self-image psychology with his best-selling book Psycho-Cybernetics. After working with hundreds of patients, he came to the conclusion that our self-image controls our behavior like a thermostat. During the winter you set your thermostat to maintain a certain temperature – let's say 70°Fahrenheit. If the temperature gets a few degrees below 70, the thermostat detects the deviation from the set goal and turns on the heating system: When the temperature reaches 70, the fire is turned off.

Your self-image works exactly the same. The picture you have in your mind is the goal your behavior is programmed to maintain.

What is your Current Self-Image?

If you believe that you are fat, unhealthy, or over weight, then that is your current self-image on yourself. **You will NEVER become "skinny" or "healthy" unless you change your self-image.** You need to change the paradigm. You can do this, it's not too late. It will take some work though. Your self-image of yourself was developed over years and years of your life and reinforced by your habits every day. That doesn't make it true though.

Here is a good test to see where your self-image is programmed: Picture yourself at the beach this summer. Do you see yourself slender, attractive, and wearing a swimsuit, or as you look now? Picture yourself one year from now. Do you see yourself being healthy and 10 pounds lighter or the same person as you are now?

If you see yourself as you are now, did you ever deviate from that image for more than a few months or weeks? Probably not. You may have gotten lean or felt healthy for 2-3 months but then you went right back to your self-image.

The way your self-image controls your behavior is by taking the form of your voice of reason. Every time you start getting better or worse results than you think you should get a voice in your head starts convincing you to go back to your old ways.

Have you ever experienced the yo-yo diet? Lose weight but then gain it back? Why do we Yo-Yo? It makes perfect sense when we realize that our self-image controls us.

This is why having a goal of losing 10 pounds is a terrible idea. Let's say you actually lose 10 pounds. Great. But if you never change your self-image to reflect the new you, you subconsciously focus on the same goal of losing 10 pounds. In order to reach "losing 10 pounds", you gain weight back, and then lose weight again) to meet your goal, but this is an endless cycle which keeps repeating itself over and over again. A much better goal would be to "lose 10 pounds and maintain my new weight while being healthy and eating a well balanced diet. Now, that's a goal!

When losing weight, you may get thoughts like:

- I've hit my calories perfectly the last two days. I've earned a cheat day.
- I think I can have another dessert today. I'll eat less tomorrow.
- Wow I'm getting too small. I should stop dieting.

You must understand that those thoughts are not yours. They are created by your old habits, trying to correct the deviation from your self-image.

How your Current Self-Image was Created?

Our mind is divided in two parts: The Conscious Mind and the Subconscious Mind. Both affect the actions of our physical body. The Conscious Mind holds your mental faculties: reason, imagination, will, memory, perception and intuition. This is the part that thinks, imagines, and makes decisions.

The Subconscious Mind has a different role. First of all it controls the functioning of the body like breathing, pumping blood, healing wounds, and so on. But it is also the place where your habits are located. The subconscious mind takes the repeated actions of the conscious mind and makes them automatic. The reason it does that is so that you can perform those actions without thinking, leaving your mental faculties free to focus on something else.

Let me give you an example you can all relate to. When you learn how to drive, all your conscious attention is focused on pressing the pedals, turning the wheel, looking in the mirrors, checking the dials – in other words making sure you don't crash. But if you repeat those actions long enough, they become subconscious and automatic. Now you probably can drive steering your knee while talking on the phone. When an action becomes subconscious your conscious attention is free to be directed on something else.

Your Self-Image is Subconscious

Your self-image is nothing but a multitude of habits and is located in the subconscious mind. It has been planted there like anything else – through repetition. If you've been exposed to an environment where people always talked about poverty and how difficult it is to earn money, through repetition those thoughts have been planted in the subconscious mind and became part of your self-image.

If you've been exposed to an environment where food is abundant and many people were overweight, through repetition those thoughts have been planted in the subconscious mind and became part of your self-image.

For example, did you know that the chances of becoming obese increase by 57% if a close friend or family member becomes obese? That's because you're constantly exposed to their way of life and ultimately that becomes your behavior as well.

How to Change your Self-Image

And finally we get to the practical part. There are two known ways to change the self-image:

- **A powerful emotional event:**
  We all heard about those people that completely changed their lives after a powerful experience. A car accident, the loss of a loved one, public humiliation, an unexpected victory, having a baby, losing your home – any of these incidents can be life-changing. But we can't control them. So instead of waiting for something like this to happen to motivate us to change our lives, we're going to use the other way.

- **Autosuggestion: Constant spaced repetition of your goal:** This is when you repeat an idea or image long enough that it is taken over by the subconscious mind and becomes your habitual way of thinking. Besides emotional shock, repetition is the only known method of influencing the subconscious mind.

For trying to lose weight, I propose two methods of autosuggestion:

1. Carrying and reading a goal card every day
2. Constantly watching videos related to success and practicing affirmations.

The Goal Card Method

The Goal Card method is simple. It involves writing your major goal on a card that you can carry loose in your pocket and reading that as many times as possible during the day. It should be read at least two times a day, before you go to sleep and right after you wake up.

The reason you carry it loose in your pocket is so you HAVE to touch it several times a day and remember your goal every time. If you put it your wallet or in a drawer you will forget about it most days. Every time you read it, the image of yourself in possession of your goal will pop up in your mind. Repeat that long enough and that image will become your self-image.

I picked up this idea from Bob Proctor and he picked it up from Napoleon Hill, the author of Think and Grow Rich the most successful personal development book of all time. Here's how Napoleon Hill explains the way the goal card works:

Any definite chief aim that is deliberately fixed in the mind and held there, with the determination to realize it, finally saturates the entire subconscious mind until it automatically influences the physical action of the body toward the attainment of that purpose.

Your definite chief aim in life should be selected with deliberate care, and after it has been selected it should be written out and placed where you will see it at least once a day, the psychological effect of which is to impress this purpose upon your subconscious mind so strongly that it accepts that purpose as a pattern or blueprint that will eventually dominate your activities in life and lead you, step by step, toward the attainment of the object back of that purpose.

Napoleon Hill explains that through constant repetition the image of your goal is taken over by the subconscious mind and it becomes your self-image. When that happens, the actions you feel like doing are those that will produce the realization of you goal. You will start acting in ways that you haven't before. In other words, instead of getting the urge to cheat and go back to your old self-image of an overweight person, you will get the urge to stick to your study plan and get to the great test taker self-image.

That's what happens when you read and carry this goal card with you long enough! The image of your goal will dominate your thoughts and your every action will be directed towards the attainment of that goal.

How my Goal Card Completely Changed my Life:

I first learned about this idea in 2012 when I was watching a video from Bob Proctor. At one point he said: "I guarantee that if you write your goal on a card, carry it in your pocket and read it at least twice a day that goal will become reality."

When most people hear this they say "Oh come on… another bullshit infomercial." But I said "Hey why not give it a shot? I'm going to write a big goal on a card and carry it with me every day for five years. If it doesn't work I don't lose anything, time will pass anyway. **But if it does work, I'm going to win BIG."**

Because I still had no idea what I wanted in life or what I enjoyed doing, I wrote down weight loss goal. I said I wanted to lose 30 pounds in 30 weeks. I'm no doctor, but I read that you can safely lose 1 pound every 1 week. Any more than that it's not healthy and probably a fad diet plan.

That goal scared the shit out of me and I couldn't see how it could possibly happen. But I kept reading the card every day. Because of my goal, 2015 ended up being the most depressing year of my life. Every day my goal card was reminding me to ACT, to START DOING SOMETHING but I was afraid and I was constantly procrastinating. I felt like a failure and with that came the feeling of guilt.

But I kept reading the card.

And…I finally achieved that goal and lost 32 pounds.

Whatever you write on the card and read every day for several months will become reality. If you don't believe me, go to YouTube and search for Earl Nightingale's "The Strangest Secret". It's about 25 minutes long but it will change your life.

How to Write your Goal Card

Now, your final objection may be that Bob/Sue down the street lost weight but you know that he/she doesn't read a goal card every day and look how fit he/she is in.

There are two kinds of people in this world that achieve outstanding success in any field:

- the unconscious competent
- those that became competent by choice and study

This person is almost certainly an unconscious competent. If you asked him why he's disciplined and committed, he probably couldn't tell you. He loves success so much that it doesn't make sense to them why other people wouldn't want to be successful.

But if you were an unconscious competent too, you wouldn't be reading this program. You need to use autosuggestion to "artificially" transform yourself into a great test taker. So you can BE YOURSELF.

Here's how my first goal card looked like:

The translation would be this:

"I'm so happy and grateful now that I am becoming fit and healthly!

In exchange for this weight loss, I offer the best services to the world I'm capable of. I eat healthy and exercise every day. I offer excellence in everything I do and I only move on to something else when I'm done with the current task. I believe in myself with all my heart and I know I can do anything I set my mind to."

That's what got me off the ground. I currently have a different goal card but the concept is the same.

You should also use these affirmations every day:

Present Tense Affirmations:

I am healthy

I exercise often

I exercise easily

I enjoy treating my body with respect

I look forward to eating healthy and natural foods

I ignore distractions

I succeed in stressful situations

Future Tense Affirmations:

I will lose my love handles

I am becoming adept at exercising and eating healthy

I am learning to enjoy becoming heathy

I will be relaxed during dieting

I will thrive under pressure

I will stay focused while eating healthy

Natural Affirmations:

Losing weight comes natural for me

Focusing feels natural to me

Dieting comes easily for me

Being healthy is enjoyable

Excising is fun

Healthy eating habits are ingrained in me

Here's how to write a goal card:

1. At the top of the card write your goal and a date by which you intend to achieve that goal. Be specific. It's not sufficient to say "I want to lose weight", you must be definite so the picture you get in your mind is clear.
2. Underneath that, write what you intend to give in return for that goal. There is no such reality as something for nothing. Your goal will be achieved at the expense of your effort.
3. Describe the conditions in which you want to achieve that goal.
4. You may place pictures of the people that inspire you at the bottom of the card (optional). I always found other people inspiring but you may be different.

Once you reach your goal you may change the goal card and set a business or personal goal instead. After all, you probably don't want losing weight or your love handles subject of your thoughts forever.

Watch videos related to losing weight

You probably heard of the idea that you are the average of the top 5 people you spend most of your time with. That's true but it doesn't necessarily mean spending time with them in real life.

If you can't surround yourself with success models in person, do it through internet videos, articles and podcasts. You will unconsciously start to act like those people. For personal success I recommend you follow any author or entrepreneur that inspires you. What I personally use is a program from Bob Proctor called 6 Minutes to Success.

This program is designed to send you short educational video every day on all important topics: personal achievement, money, relationships, education, discipline. The price is pretty high, it's 50 dollars a month but for me personally it has been invaluable. I've been in it for 2 years. You can also find many of Bob's programs for free on YouTube. For example, the Born Rich Seminar is available for free on their channel.

You can also find free YouTube videos on losing weight affirmations.

Conclusion

- The reason you fail to achieve your goals is probably your self-image
- You will never be able to maintain better results than your self-image
- To change it, you must use autosuggestion
- The forms of autosuggestion I recommend are

The goal card method

Surrounding yourself with success models in real life and online

Surrendering The Old You:

There is a way to let go of the old you in order to create a new you. You never have to be the same again. Only by choice. In order to make room for the new and reinvented you, you have to "let go" of the old you. You do this by surrendering. There is tremendous power in Surrendering.

Surrender is an important part of all spiritual practice. Ultimately it's what we're aiming to accomplish in practice. What we're surrendering to is the reality of impermanence and non-separateness. In reality, everything changes and nothing (including ourselves) is separate or self-contained. But we have deep-rooted assumptions that we exist separately from the rest of the world, that there is something in us (and others) that is permanent and static, and that happiness can be found outside of ourselves. We believe that happiness is to be found in external conditions, rather than in changing our relation to the external conditions in which we live — which is why two people can be in the same situation, with one of them happy and the other miserable. So our view of ourselves and of where happiness comes from is at odds with how things really are.

We're left with the task of realigning our views with reality, and to do that we have to surrender those views, surrender the desires that those views give rise to, and surrender the actions to which those desires give birth. And we need to accept the reality of change, non-separateness, and that things "out there" can't bring us lasting happiness.

I do not claim to be master in this subject. But please, check out the books and videos online in order to learn how to surrender.

Razor's Edge:

This single concept totally changed my life when I first learned about it in Bob Proctor's book "You Were Born Rich". I used it to advance my career and continue to use it today. I'm teaching it to my kids. It's not taught in schools…You will never hear it… Yet it is one of the most powerful mindsets you can ever have. It's a total shame that people can go their entire lives without ever knowing about it. Just learning this one concept is worth the price of this book even if you do not start eating healthy or exercising. After practicing it for more than 10 years and having huge success with it, I almost feel like I have a cheat code for life. So here it is:

You are only one inch … one step … one idea … away from turning onto the boulevard of beauty in your own life.

The line which separates winning from losing is as fine as a razor's edge… and it is! The real winners in life are, more often than not, only two or three percent more effective than those who lose. The Razor's Edge clearly illustrates this point. **You need to understand that you can be every bit as effective as anyone you read about or even hear about.** Feelings of inferiority, as well as any doubts you may be entertaining relative to your capability, will quickly fall by the wayside and be left far behind, as you near your destination.

The Razor's Edge is simply doing a little bit more … a little bit more than others … a little bit more than is expected … and a little bit more than is necessary. And it doesn't really take any special skills or talents to do it. The good news is you can have the Razor's Edge working for you. It can totally change your life. It did for me.

Vince Lombardi, former football coach of the outstanding Green Bay Packers football team, described the Razor's Edge concept in football very well when he said, "Most games are won or lost in the last two minutes of the first and second half." But what Lombardi is best remembered for—with respect to football's Razor's Edge—is the "Second Effort" concept, which he introduced for the edification of his players. In a nutshell, the "Second Effort" concept simply meant, that when a player was initially stopped by the opposing team, he would always surge forward a second time, with the added thrust of a "second effort."

Now, just consider the tremendous difference you could create in your own life if you were to adopt a similar mental attitude. For example, if you are a person who is working in sales and currently selling only three units a week, what would the consequences be for you if you were to decide to make one additional sale per week, through a conscientious application of the second effort concept?

Well, on a weekly basis, it might not appear to be a major breakthrough. However, viewed over the time frame of an entire career, it would actually amount to well over two thousand extra sales. Moreover, from a monetary standpoint, it would mean you would actually receive an extra ten years' income over the span of a forty-year career. Yes, that one sale would be the Razor's Edge difference, which could catapult you into "the big leagues" in your chosen career.

In 1947, the race horse named ARMED won $761,500. But the horse who finished second in earnings that same year won only $75,000.

Now, if you were to look at their winnings alone, it would appear that ARMED was thirteen times better than his closest competitor. However, when you compare "the times" that were actually registered by those two horses in their races, you learn that ARMED was a mere four percent better!

There was only a little difference between the two horses, but that little difference made all the difference in the world. And it's a truth I see repeated over and over again ... in every profession of life. The "greatest" golfers ... like Tiger Woods ... are only 3 or 4 strokes better than the "poorest" golfers in the tournament, but their winnings are dozens of times higher than those who come in second, third, or fourth place.

So it's rather obvious, as Bob Proctor says, "The line which separates winning from losing is as fine as a razor's edge." And he gives example after example of that very thing throughout his book, "You Were Born Rich."

The good news is you can have the Razor's Edge working for you.

It's simply doing a little bit more … a little bit more than others … a little bit more than is expected … and a little bit more than is necessary.

In Proctor's words, "One person 'just about' starts a project, the other person starts it. "One person 'just about' starts eating healthy, the other person actually started eating healthy. One individual 'almost' completes an exercise, the other does complete it. One person sees an opportunity, the other acts on it. One student 'nearly' passes the exam, the other does pass it… and although the difference in their marks may be only one percentage point out of a hundred, **it's that one point that makes all the difference."**

There's a great example in that book about the Jacobs family and how they learned how to apply this principle to their business. They were the owners of an automobile repair shop that had fallen on hard times economically … so much so they considered closing their shop. Upon interviewing them, Proctor learned that they were indeed skilled mechanics, filled with enthusiasm and confidence about the quality of their work. But they gave very little attention to the "people" part of the business.

So Proctor suggested they apply the Razor's Edge to their business … to do a little bit more. He suggested that they vacuum the inside of every car they repair, wash the outside, and make sure the windows were spotless. After all, most people don't understand very much about the mechanical aspects of a car, but people notice how a car looks and feels. About two weeks after they started applying this Razor's Edge, the Jacobs family reported having more business than ever before.

How can you get the Razor's Edge working for you?

There are dozens of things you can do. For starters,

1) Refuse to Settle for the Basics:

For example, you may have mastered the basics of reading by the fifth or sixth grade. But have you done anything since then to improve your reading skills? And you may have mastered the basics of arithmetic, but have you gone beyond that to master the skills required for saving, investing, and budgeting for your future? Get off your assets and go for something bigger and better.

2) Decide to become an expert in Something:

You see … once people understand the basics of something, they usually stop their learning in that area. Only a small percentage of people ever go on to become the acknowledged experts in a particular area. And they are the ones, of course, who typically receive the largest incomes. That's why you should look at what you're doing, and as Proctor says, ask yourself, "How good am I at doing it?" and "How much better could I be?"

3) Dedicate Your Time to Study:

All you have to do is study one hour a day in your chosen field, and in five years you will be an expert in that field. In Proctor's words, "If you were to follow this schedule rigorously, in a relatively short span of time you would stand among your peers like a giraffe in a herd of field mice."

4) Turn Your Car into A Library:

Turn your radio off and your CD player on. If you're like me, you drive thousands of miles to work or errands each year. In fact, if you drive as many as 25,000 miles per year, you're spending the equivalent of thirteen forty-hour weeks sitting behind the wheel of your car. So you've got the time to listen to educational, motivational CDs. And whether or not you consciously focus on what you're hearing, it's virtually impossible to keep on exposing your mind to good, clean, powerful, uplifting information and not be positively influenced by it. The world is filled with so much negativity it's crazy. Just listen to the crap on the evening news, it's so negative. I believe that the is a reason society tries to feed us this scarcity mindset every day. It lowers our vibrational state. If we are scared, afraid, negative, sad, we are more willing to go to that 9-5 job that we hate. We are willing to just accept a 2-week vacation. They are controlling us. Why control us? To be able to predict our behaviors... which I believe ultimately leads to getting our votes in elections. My career and personal life took off when I turned off the news and adopted an abundance mindset. There is abundance everywhere. Look for it!

5) Add the Razor's Edge Element to Your Job:

Perhaps you're in a customer service position. You will be astounded at what happens if you change your attitude towards your customers. If you tend to see customers as an interruption OF your business ... instead the reason FOR your business ... you're bound to lose some customers. But if you think of ways to sharpen your customer service skills ... and then actually do it ... you'll see an amazing difference in how you feel and in how much they buy. Try smiling at every customer. Give everyone a genuine, welcoming "hello" instead of perfunctory "hi." And make sure you go out of your way to thank them for their business.

6) Persist:

Napoleon Hill studied the greatest men and women of history to discover the secrets of their success, summarizing his findings in this book called, "Think and Grow Rich." Without a doubt, one of those secrets, he said, was persistence. On one occasion, Hill wrote, "There may be no heroic connotation to the word persistence, but the quality is to the character of man, what carbon is to steel."

Later he explained, "I had the happy privilege of analyzing both Mr. Thomas Edison and Mr. Henry Ford, year by year, over a long period of years, and therefore the opportunity to study them at close range. Therefore, I speak with actual knowledge when I say that I found no quality, save Persistence, in either of them, that even remotely suggested the major source of their stupendous achievements."

Simply put, you put the Razor's Edge to work for you when you persist, when you keep on keeping on, no matter how strenuous or challenging the course.

How can you get this to work for you?

Do one extra exercise a day, it will add up over time. Start incorporating some of the healthy food/drink choices which are listed in this book into your daily life, one by one (razor's edge), and you will soon start to see changes in your appearance and health. Does that take any special skill? No. It can totally stack the odds in your favor. I also used the Razor's Edge when I wrote my first book, which was 182 pages. I didn't write that book in one sitting. I wrote 1/2 page each day for an entire year and ended up with a complete book at the very end. Little things add up to bigger things.

What's your Razor's Edge?

Now, you may have grown up with the idea that some people have it and some people don't. Or, because some people are much better than others, they enjoy much more of the abundance of life. But I want you to understand, right here and now, this idea is absolutely false! For you are every bit as good, or as powerful, as anyone you see, know, or even hear about. Remember, since the difference between them and you is only in the area of accomplishments, and since there is something you can do that will vastly improve the results you are achieving presently, you have the potential to become even more successful than they are. You may already know how to do what others are doing (if you don't, you can learn), and since your potential power is unlimited, you can do even greater things than they are now doing.

The "something" that you must do to become more successful may not be what you think it is. But whatever it may be, rest assured, you are quite capable of doing it. You can make up in numbers what you lack in skill. Always bear in mind, however, that because each person's world is just a little bit different, the something which you must do is not necessarily the same thing the person you live with or work with, must do. Nevertheless, there is no question that you will eventually find out what it is that you must do. So make up your mind—immediately—when you do figure out what that Razor's Edge is for you, you will do it.

Now stop reading, sit back, relax, and think, really think—what is it in your life that will make the Razor's Edge difference for you? You know what it is?

Good—then do it now!

Get into the Right Mindset:

You have to get in the proper "learning" mindset and realize that this book is an opportunity to develop new skills and adopt new mindsets. No matter how hard it is at first, you'll be able to improve over time through hard work and practice. Your weight will reflect the amount of work you put in - not just your raw intelligence. Losing weight does not have to be a struggle, but a journey of learning increments filled with opportunities for growth as well as gains. You will become a better person simply by practicing the concepts in this book.

There will be a time during your dieting and exercising in which you will want to quit because you think that this is too hard in this short period of time. This is completely normal. Everyone wants to quit. You can't expect to go through this program by only going up and up and up. Success has dips. Sometimes you go up and other times you will go down. Don't judge your progress by how many pounds you are losing each day. You should instead judge yourself on the ACTION you are taking. If you ARE taking action each day, then that's how you judge your success. This phenomenon is based on the basic learning curve. At one point, the curve plateaus without ever increasing until sometime later down the road. This will seem to happen to you as you begin practicing new eating habits. Do not quit!

For some reason, the idea that you have to work every single problem correctly gets passed on from generation to generation. It's a vicious cycle. No one is perfect. Hall of Famers, the best baseball hitters of all time, only hit the ball 30% of the time (3 out of 10 times at bat). That's what a batting average of 300 means. Conversely, this means they failed 70% of the time. Think about it. The best hitters in history never hit the ball in 7 out of 10 at bats. Don't pressure yourself for perfection, keep it all in perspective. In basketball, you have to shoot 50% to be considered an average player. If you make an extra 10 shots per hundred, you are an All-Star. In real life, the odds are a little different. You don't have to be right every time. In fact, it doesn't matter how many times you strike out. In life, to be a success, you only have to be right once. It doesn't matter how many failed diets you have been on in the past. You only have to on one diet that succeeds in the NOW, and you will win!

Don't be afraid to fail. Examples of great men and women failing have become emblematic of success: Michael Jordan, the greatest basketball player in the history of the game (sorry Kobe) missed over 9,000 shots in his career and he lost almost 300 games. 26 times he's been trusted to take the game-winning shot and missed. He failed over and over and over again in his life. And that is why he succeeded. Babe Ruth struck out 1,335 times to get his near record 714 home runs. Thomas Edison persisted through 1,300 failed experiments until he finally invented the light bulb. Abraham Lincoln lost over 90% of the debates his participated in; but he is still considered the best of any president. If you read the biography of any famous actor, you will learn that they did not get the role more often than they did land the role. The best comedians of all time; Richard Prior, Steven Kinison, bombed on stage more often, at least in the beginning, than they killed it. True victory is preceded by defeat.

Doesn't matter how many times you failed before. If you focus, visualize your goal, and avoid the naysayers, success will come. You only have to be right one time. As you work through your mistakes, it is like swinging a machete through a thick vegetated forest. You are creating new pathways that didn't exist before. As you eat healthy and exercise, you are forcing yourself to learn new skills by creating new pathways and connections. Once you create the new pathway, it's always there. This is the law of

Averages. In order to double your success rate, you will have start doubling your failure rate. That's the only way to do it.

Visualize your goal and stay focused. Do something healthy a little bit each day. Exercise in the morning, at lunch time, and at night. When you start gaining momentum a little bit each day, a compounding effect starts happening. Since compounding is an exponential function, it will seem to get easier and you will be amazed by how much material you have gone through. Even on days where you are the most tired and don't feel like exercising, try to do just one thing to improve yourself by 1%. Improving yourself by just 1% per day for one month is not 30% better... it is much more than that because of the compounding effect.

Consider this question:

How many times would you have to fold regular size loose leaf paper in order to reach the moon? 42 times, 150 times, 275,000 times?

The mean (average) distance from the Earth is about 384,000 km, or about 3.84×10^{12} pages away. So you'd expect that you'll need an awful lot of foldings to get there, right? Paper folding is *exponential*, so that if you fold it one time, it becomes 2 pages thick. If you fold it three times, it will be 6 pages thick. If you fold it a fourth time, it'll be 16 pages thick, a fifth time will be 32 pages thick, and so on. By the time you get to 9 foldings, the folded paper is bigger than the original ream of 500 sheets. By the time you get to 20 foldings, the folded paper is more than 10 kilometers high, which surpasses Mt. Everest! 41 foldings will get slightly more than halfway to the Moon, so that means that 42 foldings is all it takes! That's the power of an exponential.

The point is this: **Radical changes can happen in small steps.** Small things turn into huge things by simply compounding what you have over and over again. Not only is this a powerful concept in personal finance, but in everything that you do. Albert Einstein called "compounding" the most powerful force in the universe. The same affect happens when you study. The more you eat healthy and exercise, the easier it becomes. The more time you spend studying, the perception of time will start flying by and the task becomes easier and more manageable. Things are rarely harder than they first appear.

Most people only use a fraction, maybe 5 or 10%, of their potential. It's time to tap into the other 95%. Whether or not you choose to find the time to exercise is entirely up to you.

Vacuum Law of Prosperity:

The universe creates a vacuum. In order to receive something new, you first have to get rid of something. This is essentially Newton's 3rd Law. But you need to make room for it to show up in your life. The universe has no choice; it will show up. But first, you will have to make room for it to manifest. You want to lose weight? Well, you have to get rid of some of your current (large) clothes in your closet...in order to make room for your new (smaller) clothes to show it. Clean out your junk food drawer in order to make room for the new healthy food choices to show up. Get rid of the carbonated drinks to make room for the lemon water and green tea to show up. Want to start a side business? Well, the first step is to clear off a small area of your desk at home, buy a small cabinet drawer and some manila folders for your new project. Label it "new project". This new area creates room for it to manifest… and it will. It all starts with the first step.

80/20 principle:

The overall strategy that I recommend is based on the 80/20 principle. The 80/20 principle is named after the Italian economist Vilfredo Pareto, who observed that 80% of income in Italy was received by 20% of the Italian population. The assumption is that most of the results in any situation are determined by a small number of causes and that 80 percent of your outcomes come from 20 percent of your inputs. There are business examples such as 20 percent of employees are responsible for 80 percent of a company's output or 20 percent of customers are responsible for 80 percent of the revenues. You may also notice how you may only wear 20% of the clothes in your closet 80% of the time.

The important thing to understand is that in your life there are certain activities you do (your 20 percent) that account for the majority (your 80 percent) of your happiness and outputs. When you start to analyze and breakdown your life into elements it's very easy to see 80/20 ratios all over the place. The trick, once your key happiness determinants have been identified, is to make everything work in harmony and avoid wasting time on those 80 percent activities that produce little satisfaction for you.

The message is simple enough – **focus on activities that produce the best outcomes for you.**

Many people trying to lose weight do not get results because they waste time by having poor choices. Sure, they did their exercises during the day, eat healthy at morning and lunch, and then drink 4 beers at night time. Focus on the results and making right choices.

What causes Love Handles?

Many people give thought to the reason they have love handles. Some wonder if they were destined to have a bigger stomach or if their body is just built that way. It's a better option to stop feeling sorry for yourself and face facts. The most common cause of love handles is an unhealthy diet. No one is more responsible for love handles than ourselves.

Some people may have a higher metabolism than others but your body can still be controlled by you. Don't treat yourself every weekend if you don't have a great metabolism, a moderate treat would not harm much. Once you understand the reason you have love handles it may be possible for you to control them. They're caused by extra fat around the abdomen, an accumulation of subcutaneous fat below the skin.

Another layer known as visceral fat lies deep inside the body and is close to our vital organs, some of that is necessary to protect our organs and the rest is hard to get rid of. You can decrease both types of fat by maintaining a healthy diet and lifestyle which will help you avoid love handles.

Lack of exercise is another common cause of love handles. Someone who exercises regularly has a much lower chance of having love handles. Your hormones get re-balanced and your metabolic rate is increased by exercise, which helps to burn those love handles. Many overdo the cardio which is not advisable or necessary. Regular exercise changes our body, increases confidence, and makes us feel good.

Saying good riddance to love handles may not be an easy task in most cases, but it shouldn't be too much of a tall order either. Love handles will pose a dangerous capability of going obese, along with being unnecessarily uncomfortable in your quest of attaining that perfect figure that you have been hunting for.

How to Prevent Accumulation of Fat around the Belly?

- Avoid eating white rice and sugary supplements.
- Avoid consuming red meat and junk foods.
- Walk at least 1 kilometer on a daily basis.
- Eat green vegetables and fruits.
- Lower down the sodium intake.
- Skipping rope can be a very good exercise to keep belly in shape.
- Avoid taking stress.
- Do cardio exercises.

Here are over 50 home remedies for getting rid of love handles and each of them will call for some dedication and commitment before they bear fruit. Start incorporating some of these into your daily life, one by one (razor's edge), and you will soon start to see changes in your appearance and health.

Home Remedies for Love Handles

1.Drink Plenty of Water

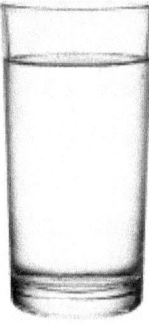

Water is life and it is essential to your good health. The earth is made up of 70% water. Drinking two glasses of hot or warm water a half to two hours prior to meals is a good way to keep belly fat under check. You should also consider drinking the advised eight glasses of water a day to help optimize body metabolism and avoid chances of overeating. The amount of water people need per day is up for debate, but studies suggest adults need nine to 16 cups. However, this number varies depending on activity level, age, and how much water people are consuming in coffee, tea, or water-rich veggies and fruit. Here's how to keep yourself hydrated: Begin by drinking a glass of water as soon as you wake up, and 35 minutes before eating any big meal. This will help control appetite, too. Get in the habit of keeping a water bottle on hand at all times. And if the taste beings to bore, spice up the taste buds with a squeeze of citrus to the glass! Before you know it, all the benefits of water will be right at your fingertips and in your body.

Certain toxins in the body can cause the skin to inflame, which results in clogged pores and acne. While science saying water makes the skin wrinkle free is contradictory, water *does* flush out these toxins and can reduce the risk of pimples. Our kidneys process 200 quarts of blood daily, sifting out waste and transporting urine to the bladder. Yet, kidneys need enough fluids to clear away what we don't need in the body. In order to really focus, a glass of water could help people concentrate and stay refreshed and alert. Water can also help fight those tired eyes too . One of the most common symptoms of dehydration is tiredness.

2. Minimize Stress

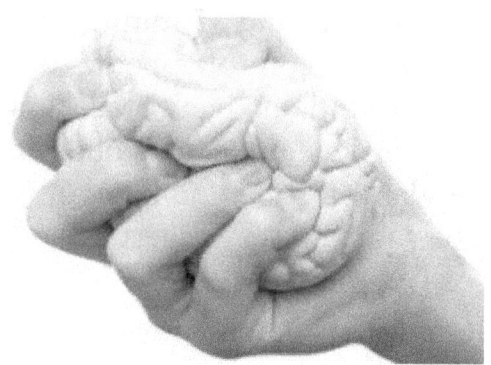

Stress has negative health consequences and will add up to fat accumulation in the body. Stress leads to the breakdown of muscle mass and increases fat content and this keeping it far from reach will help eliminate this fat. Practice basic stress management skills to avoid this negative state and add up one more arsenals for fat elimination of such fat.

Relax. You deserve it, it's good for you, and it takes less time than you think. You don't need a spa weekend or a retreat. All you have to do is meditate. A few minutes of practice per day can help ease anxiety. Research suggests that daily meditation may alter the brain's neural pathways, making you more resilient to stress. It's simple. Sit up straight with both feet on the floor. Close your eyes. Focus your attention on reciting -- out loud or silently -- a positive mantra such as "I feel at peace" or "I love myself." Place one hand on your belly to sync the mantra with your breaths. Let any distracting thoughts float by like clouds.

Slow down and be Present. Take 5 minutes and focus on only one behavior with awareness. Notice how the air feels on your face when you're walking and how your feet feel hitting the ground. Enjoy the texture and taste of each bite of food. When you spend time in the moment and focus on your senses, you should feel less tense.

3. Drinking Lemon Water

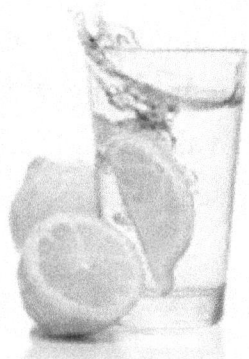

Vitamin C is like our immune system's jumper cables, and lemon juice is full of it. The level of vitamin C in your system is one of the first things to plummet when you're stressed, which is why experts recommended popping extra vitamin C during especially stressful days. As already mentioned, lemons are high in potassium, which is good for heart health, as well as brain and nerve function. It helps flush out the toxins in your body by enhancing enzyme function, stimulating your liver. Lemons contain pectin fiber, which assists in fighting hunger cravings.

The biggest lemon water benefit may be from the temperature of the water and not even the added lemon.

Drinking any water, or especially warm water, first thing in the morning can help flush the digestive system and rehydrate the body. Lemon water has been cited as a remedy for numerous skin and internal remedies and among them slimming procedures. Drinking lemon water is an effective way to detoxify the liver and allow it to work more efficiently on fats thus rid your belly of stagnating fat levels. Have a single lemon fruit and a glass of preferably hot drinking water early in the morning. Squeeze out the juice and take it every day on waking up then spend thirty minutes before eating anything else.

4. Get Enough Sleep

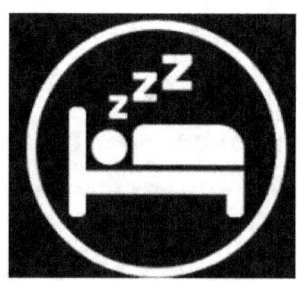

Even if you eat the exact same diet as your friend, if you're not getting the sleep your body needs, you won't drop as much fat as them. A recent study from the University of Chicago compared the weight-loss results from sleeping eight and a half hours per night versus only five and a half hours per night.

The body requires enough sleep to optimize its working and respond to hormones effectively. Lack of sleep levels will inhibit the body's response to insulin and thus heighten fat deposition which increases with more fat being stored around the waist line. Having at least seven hours of sound and continuous sleep every day is a good way to restore your energy and allow the body to function optimal.

Sleeping in won't make you fat. In fact, a new study shows that more hours in the sack could help you slim down by reducing how much control your genes have on your weight. The study, published in the journal *Sleep*, looked at the sleep patterns and body mass index (BMI) of over 1,000 twins. On average, the people in the study slept 7.2 hours a night, which falls within the National Sleep Foundation's recommended seven to nine hours.

5.Fish Oil

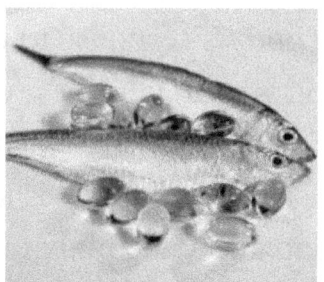

Eating fish rich in omega-3 fats is a great way to accelerate body metabolism and speed up fat oxidation. Most of the sea animals along with their products contain this vital component that helps speed up this process. Simply eat such fish three times every week or use their oils for every day recipes and you are good to go. Fish and fish oil contain omega-3 acids responsible for fat digestion and reduction of fat deposition along the waistline. For persons who may not like fish oil they can turn to fish as a source of the acids. Consuming a whole teaspoonful of fish oil every day is a good way to harness the benefits of these oils or alternatively eat omega-rich fish such salmon every three days for good results.

Also, it's been proven to aid the body in weight loss, fertility, healthy pregnancy, healthy skin and increased energy. Most of the health benefits of fish oil are because it is one of natures' richest sources of omega-3 fatty acids like Docosahexaenoic acid (DHA) and Eicosapentaenoic acid (EPA).

6.Tomatoes

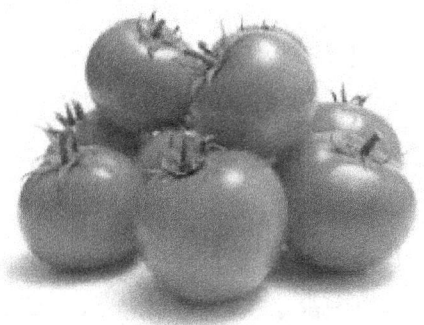

Eating raw tomatoes also helps in reducing the belly fat. Tomatoes are also an excellent source vitamin C, biotin, molybdenum and vitamin K. They are also a very good source of copper, potassium, manganese, dietary fiber, vitamin A (in the form of beta-carotene), vitamin B6, folate, niacin, vitamin E and phosphorus. The many health benefits of tomatoes can be attributed to their wealth of nutrients and vitamins, including an impressive amount of vitamins A, C, and K, as well as significant amounts of vitamin B6, folate, and thiamin. Tomatoes are also a good source of potassium, manganese, magnesium, phosphorous, and copper

Tomatoes are widely known for their outstanding antioxidant content, including, of course, their oftentimes-rich concentration of lycopene. Researchers have recently found an important connection between lycopene, its antioxidant properties, and bone health. A study was designed in which tomato and other dietary sources of lycopene were removed from the diets of postmenopausal women for a period of 4 weeks, to see what effect lycopene restriction would have on bone health. At the end of 4 weeks, women in the study started to show increased signs of oxidative stress in their bones and unwanted changes in their bone tissue. The study investigators concluded that removal of lycopene-containing foods (including tomatoes) from the diet was likely to put women at increased risk of osteoporosis. They also argued for the importance of tomatoes and other lycopene-containing foods in the diet. We don't always think about antioxidant protection as being important for bone health, but it is, and tomato lycopene (and other tomato antioxidants) may have a special role to play in this area.

7.Beans

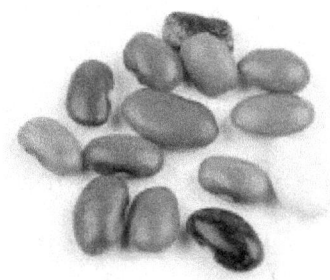

Beans provide more of soluble fiber to reduce belly fat along with provision of bacteria activity along the gut. Adding a small quantity of beans to daily meals preferably for dinner is a simple way to fight off the belly fat. Beans can be the least expensive source of protein, especially when compared to fresh meat. Aside from protein, complex carbs and fiber, beans contain a powerhouse of nutrients including antioxidants, and vitamins and minerals, such as copper, folate, iron, magnesium, manganese, phosphorous, potassium and zinc.

Studies have shown that people who eat more legumes have a lower risk of heart disease, and the phytochemicals found in beans might be partially to thank, since they protect against it. Beans contain a wide range of cancer-fighting plant chemicals, specifically, isoflavones and phytosterols which are associated with reduced cancer risk. Beans provide the body with soluble fiber, which plays an important role in controlling blood cholesterol levels. Studies find that about 10 grams of soluble fiber a day—the amount in 1/2 to 1 1/2 cups of navy beans—reduces LDL cholesterol by about 10 percent. Beans also contain saponins and phytosterols, which help lower cholesterol.

8. Eating Vitamin C Rich Foods

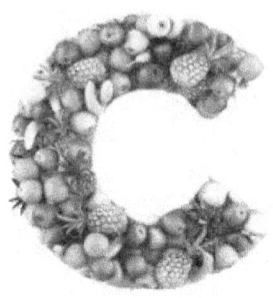

These micro-nutrients are important in fat metabolism so the body utilizes the available fat deposits. Eating a fruit every day is a good way to tap into this immense potential Vitamin C is probably best known as an antioxidant. This is a word that we use frequently but don't always stop to think about in terms of its meaning. Antioxidants are forms of molecules that help keep chemical reactions in our body in check. In particular, antioxidants help prevent excessive activity on the part of free radical molecules. (Free radicals are forms of molecules that tend to be very reactive, and too many free radicals in the wrong place at the wrong time can do damage to our cells and tissue.) Vitamin C and other antioxidants help prevent that damage. Damage to the lens of the eye, damage to molecules circulating around in our bloodstream, and damage to genetic material (DNA) in our cells are all examples of damage that have been shown to be prevented under certain circumstances by vitamin C.

One interesting application of vitamin C as an antioxidant is its ability to transform iron into a state that is better absorbed in the intestine. Including vitamin C-rich foods in recipes with your best iron sources can potentially be a way to enhance iron absorption.

9.Taking Cranberry Juice

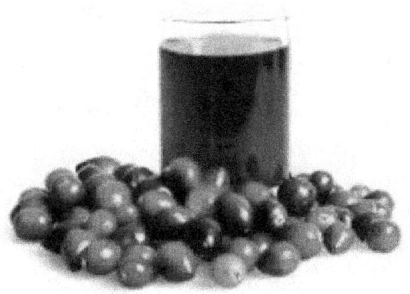

Cranberries provide a rich source of organic acids needed as digestive enzymes. The fats under this category are vital for emulsification of certain fats that may not be easy for assimilation by the body. Mix a cup of unsweetened cranberry juice with a cup of water and drink a cup early in the morning. You can also consider having a share of the juice at each of the major meals for effective results.

The health benefits of cranberry juice include relief from urinary tract infection, respiratory disorders, kidney stones, cancer, and heart disease. It is also beneficial in preventing stomach disorders and diabetes, as well as gum diseases caused by dental plaque. Phytonutrients, which are naturally derived plant compounds, are present in cranberries and have been found to prevent a wide range of health problems.

Cranberries are a versatile fruit and their benefits make them useful in food as well as in medicinal products. The Latin name for cranberry plant is *Vaccinium macrocarpon* and it is one of the native fruits of North America. Cranberries have a tremendous amount of antioxidant capacity as compared to other fruits and vegetables like broccoli, spinach, and apples. One cup of cranberries offers a total 8983 antioxidant capacity.

10. Dairy Products

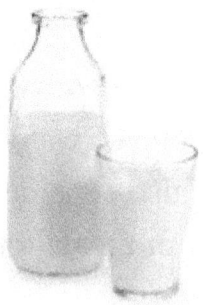

Milk products especially milk, yoghurt and cheese supply calcium that is needed to keep your fat levels low. Adding some small quantities to daily meals will help keep calcitriol under minimal levels. This hormone is responsible for accumulation of body fat and as such putting it to the lowest ebb will help combat growth of belly fat.

Milk and dairy foods are healthy foods and considered nutrient-rich because they serve as good sources of calcium and vitamin D as well as protein and other essential nutrients. They provide phosphorus, potassium, magnesium, and vitamins A, B12, and riboflavin[1].

The calcium in milk, yogurt, and cheese is significant yet most people don't get enough calcium or vitamin D each day. Getting the recommended three servings of dairy per day can help build bone mass, leading to improved bone health throughout the life cycle.

11. Minimize Consumption of Carbonated Drinks

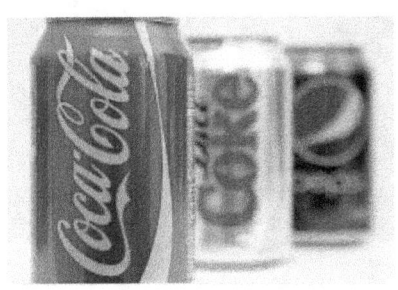

While these drinks are common place in society, their fun stops with the increase in abdominal fat due to the sugar levels spiking your appetite. Taking alternative drinks such as fresh fruit juice will help you avoid these sugars and the consequential effects on your dieting habits which boost your war on belly fat. Coke and other carbonated drinks contain the gas carbon dioxide.

When you drink Coke, you swallow both liquid and gas bubbles. A lot of the time you release this gas with a quick belch. Though not a very polite thing to do, belching lets gas escape from your body. However, in some cases drinking a lot of Coke can cause bloated or gassy feelings in the stomach and digestive tract. Coke contains sugar, water and carbon dioxide infused into the liquid. Opening a can of coke allows the compressed carbon dioxide to form bubbles and escape into the air. The bubbly, fizzy feeling of Coke in your mouth partly comes from the bubbles of CO2. Lots of the gas escapes from your mouth or resurfaces from your throat as a belch. However, drinking lots of Coke at one time forces large amounts of the liquid into your stomach where the gas may pass to your intestines.

12. Eliminate Junk Foods in Your Diet

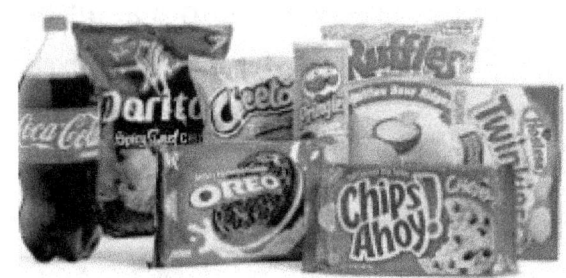

These types of food are known as junk food. They are foods that are high in calories, low in nutrients and usually contain harmful synthetic chemicals. Most junk foods are processed food; thus, they are no longer in their natural state. In addition, they are stripped of certain essential nutrients. Foods with little or no nutritional value tend to have more impact on fat storage in the body and it's only wise that you raise a red flag on them and flush them out. Such include sugars, junk foods and salt. Replacing commonplace non-nutritional value with vegetables and other valuable products in your diet will help you shape your belly and eliminate the extra fat camping in those sensitive regions.

Junk food plays a major role in the obesity epidemic. By the year 2050, the rate of obesity in the U.S. is expected to reach 42 percent, according to researchers at Harvard University. Children who eat fast food as a regular part of their diets consume more fat, carbohydrates and processed sugar and less fiber than those who do not eat fast food regularly. Junk food in these children's diets accounts for 187 extra calories per day, leading to 6 additional pounds of weight gain per year. Obesity increases your risk for cardiovascular disease, diabetes and many other chronic health conditions.

10. Green Tea Benefits

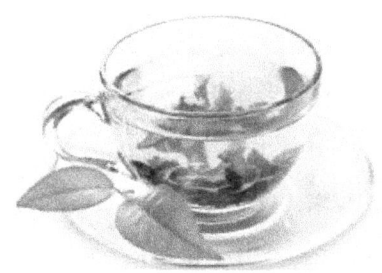

Green tea helps you strike a balance between optimization of body metabolism and appetite so you don't have too much of fat to store around. You may choose to overhaul your drinks cabinet and replace it with this tea or simply introduce it along your loved meals that are healthy. There are numerous studies on the benefit of green tea. A study published in the American journal of nutrition reckoned that persons who had four cups of this tea on a daily period indicated a fat loss of up to six pounds over a period of two months. Green tea contains a component known as EGCG which is known to boost metabolism and thus reduce the fat content in one's body. One needs to add a few leaves of green tea or the tea bag to hot water and cover it for five to ten minutes. Strain the mixture and top up with honey for tasting then serve.

Green tea is the healthiest beverage on the planet. It is loaded with antioxidants and nutrients that have powerful effects on the body. This includes improved brain function, fat loss, a lower risk of cancer and many other incredible benefits. Here are 10 health benefits of green tea that have been confirmed in human research studies. Green tea is more than just green liquid. Many of the bioactive compounds in the tea leaves do make it into the final drink, which contains large amounts of important nutrients. It is loaded with polyphenols like flavonoids and catechins, which function as powerful antioxidants. These substances can reduce the formation of free radicals in the body, protecting cells and molecules from damage. These free radicals are known to play a role in aging and all sorts of diseases. One of the more powerful compounds in green tea is the antioxidant Epigallocatechin Gallate (EGCG), which has been studied to treat various diseases and may be one of the main reasons green tea has such powerful medicinal properties. Green tea also has small amounts of minerals that are important for health. Try to choose a higher quality brand of green tea, because some of the lower quality brands can contain excessive levels of fluoride

11. Add Lime to Your Drinking Water

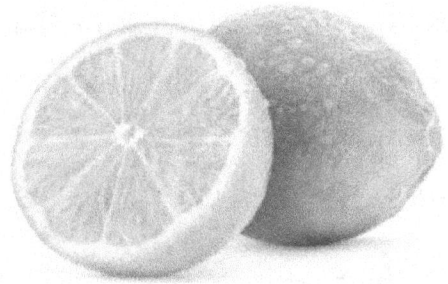

Though having plenty of water every day will help your body work out to perfect position, adding a spoonful of lime to each of the glasses will produce excellent results in most circumstances. It's preferable to have the lime with warm water as this is faster in its working to detoxify the body and speed up the rate of metabolism for fat elimination on love handles. Besides, it tastes delicious!

Lime is very well-known as a cure for scurvy, the disease which is caused from a deficiency of vitamin-C. It is characterized by frequent infections that show as normal cold symptoms, cracked lips and lip corners, ulcers on the tongue and in the mouth. You can also spot scurvy from spongy, swollen and bleeding gums. Since its cause is a deficiency of vitamin-C, its remedy is none other than vitamin-C, and lime is full of this this essential vitamin. In the past, soldiers and sailors were given lime to keep them safe from scurvy, which was a horrible and potentially fatal disease back then. Even now, it is distributed among the workers working in polluted environments like furnaces, painting shops, heat treatments, cement factories, mines, and other dangerous work environments to protect them from scurvy.

Skin Care: Lime juice and its natural oils are very beneficial for skin when consumed orally or applied externally. It rejuvenates the skin, keeps it shining, protects it from infections and reduces body odor due to the presence of a large amount of vitamin-C and Flavonoids. Those are both class-1 anti-oxidants, and have antibiotic and disinfectant properties. When applied externally on skin, its acids scrub out the dead cells, cures dandruff, rashes, and bruises. It can also be used to create a refreshing bathing experience if its juice or oil is mixed into your bathing water.

12. Have Figs in Your Daily Diets

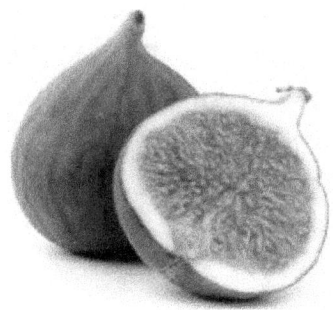

The fig tree is a member of mulberry family. The health benefits of figs come from the presence of minerals, vitamins and fiber contained in the fruit. Figs contain a wealth of beneficial nutrients, including vitamin A, vitamin B1, vitamin B2, calcium, iron, phosphorus, manganese, sodium, potassium and chlorine. Figs are a rich source of calcium, potassium, iron and fiber along with numerous vitamins including vitamin B1, B2 and vitamin A that are essential for optimal body working. Fiber helps in digestion and slows sugar absorption which aids in keeping fat accumulation in check. One can have a few of these as dry fruit on a daily basis for better results.

Although dried figs are available throughout the year, there is nothing like the unique taste and texture of fresh figs. They are lusciously sweet with a texture that combines the chewiness of their flesh, the smoothness of their skin, and the crunchiness of their seeds. California figs are available from June through September; some European varieties are available through autumn.

Figs grow on the Ficus tree (Ficus carica), which is a member of the Mulberry family. They are unique in that they have an opening, called the "ostiole" or "eye," which is not connected to the tree, but which helps the fruit's development by increasing its communication with the environment. Figs range dramatically in color and subtly in texture depending upon the variety. The majority of figs are dried, either by exposure to sunlight or through an artificial process, creating a sweet and nutritious dried fruit that can be enjoyed throughout the year.

13. Chia Seeds

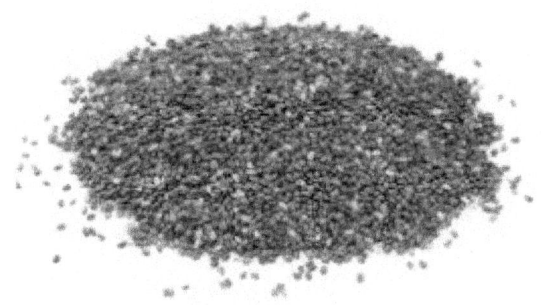

Chia seeds are a great source of the omega-3 fats that help avoid accumulation of fats around the belly. These seeds provide a good amount of these fats along with other antioxidants that adds to the general improvement of your health. Having a single spoonful of these seeds on a daily basis is good enough for the desired results.

To top things off, chia seeds are a "whole grain" food, are usually grown organically, are non-GMO and naturally free of gluten. Bottom Line: Despite their tiny size, chia seeds are among the most nutritious foods on the planet. They are loaded with fiber, protein, Omega-3 fatty acids and various micronutrients. Another area where chia seeds shine is in their high amount of antioxidants. These antioxidants protect the sensitive fats in the seeds from going rancid Although antioxidant *supplements* are not very effective, getting antioxidants from *foods* can have positive effects on health. Most importantly, antioxidants fight the production of free radicals, which can damage molecules in cells and contribute to ageing and diseases like cancer.

14. Ginger Tea

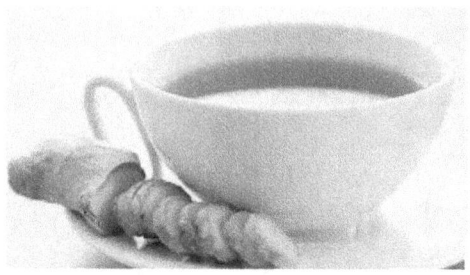

Ginger apart from being a digestive facilitator also acts as a thermogenic component and is one of the most trusted among the effective home remedies to lose belly fat. This component raises the body temperature which is essential for facilitating the combustion of body fat. Mix four cups of hot water with a single spoon of honey, ginger and lemon for effective remedy then have a cup of this tea each morning.

Ginger has anti-inflammatory properties and thus may help relieve muscle soreness after exercise, according to a study published in "The Journal of Pain" in 2010. Subjects participated in weight-training exercise to induce muscle pain and were then given either raw ginger, heated ginger or a placebo. Researchers observed pain intensity over the following three days and found that participants who took raw or heated ginger experienced less pain than those who took the placebo. Therefore, drinking ginger tea after tough workouts may help you cope with exercise-related muscle soreness.

15. Garlic

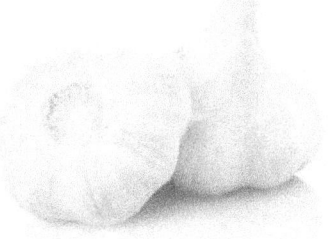

Garlic has some of the best known anti-obesity properties that make it a good bet for reducing fat belly. Garlic helps inhibit the process of fat generation and deposition by body cells and thus restricts the accumulation of fat in the body. One can simply add garlic to their meals but a more efficient way involves eating raw garlic for better results. Garlic is a plant in the onion family, grown for its cooking properties and health effects. It is high in a sulfur compound called Allicin, which is believed to bring most of the health benefits.

Garlic may help improve your iron metabolism. That's because the daily sulfides in garlic can help increase production of a protein called ferroportin. (Ferroportin is a protein that runs across the cell membrane, and it forms a passageway that allows stored iron to leave the cells and become available where it is needed.) In addition to being a good source of selenium, garlic may be a more reliable source as well. Garlic is what scientists call a "seleniferous" plant: it can uptake selenium from the soil even when soil concentrations do not favor this uptake.

16. Dandelion Tea

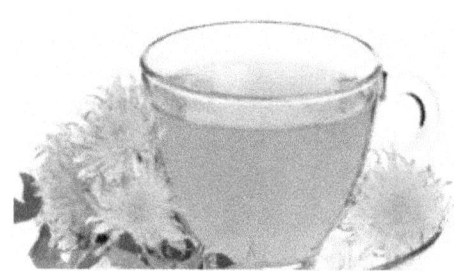

Dandelion is effective against fat accumulation in the belly caused by water retention. Dandelion just like lemon accelerates the liver metabolism thereby improving on its capacity to oxidize most of the fats. A teaspoonful of crushed dandelion root mixed with mint leaves, ginger, honey and water in specific proportions will taste good for drinking. Having two to four cups a day is a good ratio in most cases.

The compounds in the root "stimulate digestion, increase bile flow and can act as mild laxatives," says naturopath Dr. Robert Kachko, ND, LAc. This part of the dandelion works on regulating the liver and stimulating digestion. "Most conditions of the liver/gallbladder can have a use for dandelion root, but it should be prescribed by someone with training," cautions Kachko. The leaf is used to treat ailments of the kidneys; its chief function is as a diuretic. However, unlike prescription medication, it is high in potassium -- so it replenishes lost electrolytes immediately. According to Memorial Sloan-Kettering Cancer Center's Integrative Medicine Service, studies have shown dandelion to lower blood sugar levels overall. When used for help with bloating, dandelion tea has been shown have a significant effect on water content in the body because of its diuretic properties.

17. Cinnamon

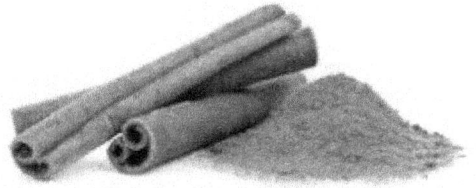

Cinnamon is one of the most delicious and healthiest spices on the planet. It can lower blood sugar levels, reduce heart disease risk factors, and has a plethora of other impressive health benefits. Cinnamon is a thermogenic that helps reduce the overall body fat along with belly fat. Spicing your meals and beverages with a spoonful of cinnamon powder is a good way to use cinnamon.

Even if you do not suffer from diabetes, you may want to include cinnamon in your diet for many of the same reasons as those who do. Cinnamon has been proven to fight fungal, bacterial, and viral elements in foods, thus preventing spoilage. It's no surprise that in the Middle Ages, when food spoilage was far more frequent due to lack of refrigeration, many recipes, both sweet and savory, were flavored with the spice. But these properties of cinnamon do not extend merely to the foods cinnamon seasons. Consumers of cinnamon can benefit from these properties as well, according to our experts, who say cinnamon can be used as part of a treatment for anything from lung problems to the common cold.

18. Lean Meat

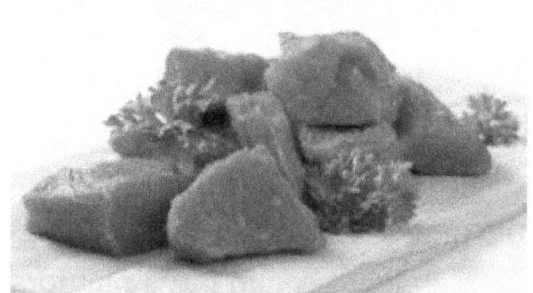

Protein is a highly thermogenic food element and thus including it in your daily diet is a good way to accelerate fat burning. Since animal proteins work more effectively than vegetable based proteins, eating lean meat will add to the numerous benefits of these substances.

Health benefits of lean meat. Lean meats are a good source of protein and have fewer calories than non-lean meats. Lean meats are popular amongst people following low calorie and low fat diets. Poultry is a good source of selenium, vitamins B3 and B6, and choline. Lean meats, such as chicken, turkey, and fish, are often touted as being essential for good health due to their small amounts of dietary fat. But the low fat content is not the only reason why these meats can improve your health. Lean meats have been found to be able to effectively help you achieve weight loss, prevent falls, and keep your hair and nails looking shiny and healthy. With these healthy benefits, lean meats should be on the top of your shopping list.

19. Hot Peppers

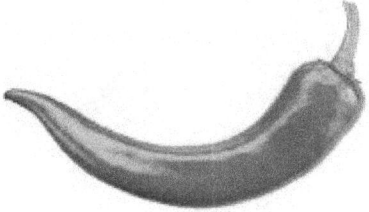

Whether you love hot peppers or can't take the heat, here's some interesting intel about the fiery produce: They can protect your heart. The health benefit comes from capsaicin (pronounced kap-say-sin), the same compound that makes chili peppers like cayennes, jalapenos, and habaneros so hot. Hot pepper has capsaicin, which is known to have thermogenic properties. Spicing daily meals with hot peppers whether raw, cooked, powdered or dry is a great way to harness the underlying potential in stimulating fat metabolism. Peppers have a lot going for them. They're low in calories and are loaded with good nutrition. All varieties are excellent sources of vitamins A and C, potassium, folic acid, and fiber. Plus, the spicy ones liven up bland food, making it more satisfying. Peppers come in all sizes and colors. Some pack heat. Others are sweet. You can get them fresh, frozen, dried, or canned.

20. Coconut Oil

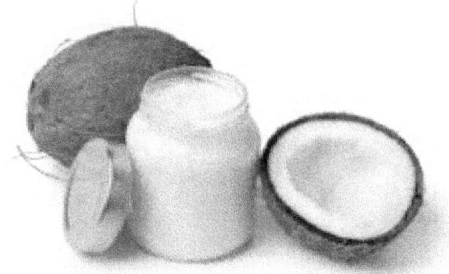

Coconut oil is high in natural saturated fats. Saturated fats not only increase the healthy cholesterol (known as HDL) in your body, but also help to convert the LDL "bad" cholesterol into good cholesterols. By Increasing the HDL's in the body, it helps promote heart health, and lower the risk of heart disease.

Coconut oil has some good effects on the rate of metabolism along with being composed of medium chain fatty acids that are easier to digest. This oil helps speed up the rate of metabolism for elimination of fat. Completely replacing your oils with this one is a good way to avoid increases in belly fat. Coconut oil has a multitude of health benefits, which include but are not limited to skin care, hair care, improving digestion and immunity against a host of infections and diseases. The oil is used not just in tropical countries, where coconut plantations are abundant, but also in the US and the UK. People are discovering the wonders this oil can create and it is again gaining popularity throughout the world. Let us see how many of these benefits you are aware of.

21. Cucumber

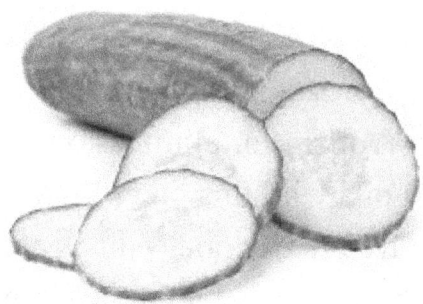

Cucumbers are rich in silicon and sulfur, which are good facilitators for fat combustion. Combining lemon with cucumber is an effective way to turn round the balance and shed off the fat in your belly. Eating a slice of cucumber with each meal along with lemon juice is recommended for standard practice.

Cucumbers are good sources of phytonutrients (plant chemicals that have protective or disease preventive properties) such flavonoids, lignans and triterpenes, which have antioxidant, anti-inflammatory and anti-cancer benefits, according to World's Healthiest Foods. The peel and seeds are the most nutrient-dense parts of the cucumber. They contain fiber and beta-carotene, a form of vitamin A that is good for eyes, reports Livestrong.com. A study published in the Pakistan Journal of Nutrition found that cucumber seeds were a good source of minerals, and contained calcium.

22. Apple Cider Vinegar

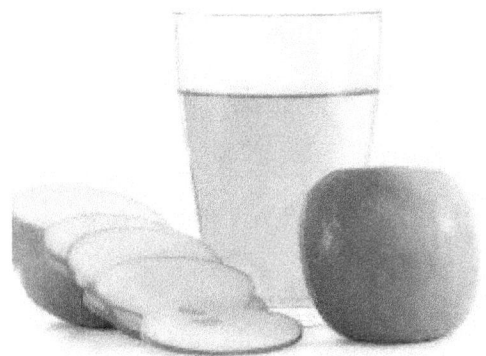

Apple cider vinegar has acidic and corrosive properties that make it a good element for assimilation of proteins used in the production of hormones and enzymes. Adding a spoonful of ACV to a glass of water for drinking is an easy way to tap into this potential.

While the uses for white vinegar are plentiful, apple cider vinegar has arguably even more applications. Its wide-ranging benefits (rivaling the number of uses for tea tree oil and other nifty natural helpers) include everything from curing hiccups to alleviating cold symptoms, and some people have turned to apple cider vinegar to help with health concerns including diabetes, cancer, heart problems, high cholesterol, and weight issues.

23. Honey

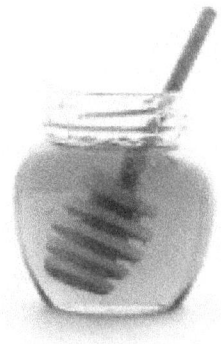

Honey contains a treasure chest of hidden nutritional and medicinal value for centuries. The sweet golden liquid from the beehive is a popular kitchen staple loaded with antibacterial and antifungal properties that has been used since the early days of Egyptian tombs. Honey's scientific super powers contribute to its vastly touted health benefits for the whole body. The healthy natural sweetener offers many nutritional benefits depending on its variety. Raw honey is the unpasteurized version of commonly used honey and only differs in its filtration, which helps extend its shelf life. A tablespoon of raw honey contains 64 calories, is fat-free, cholesterol-free, and sodium-free, says the National Honey Board. Its composition is roughly 80 percent carbohydrates, 18 percent water, and two percent vitamins, minerals, and amino acids.

Take a medium glass and fill it with hot water. Add the juice of 1 lemon and 1 tablespoon of honey to it. Drink this after waking up in the morning as a first thing. Practice this remedy on a regular basis and you will certainly notice the difference.

24. Hot Water

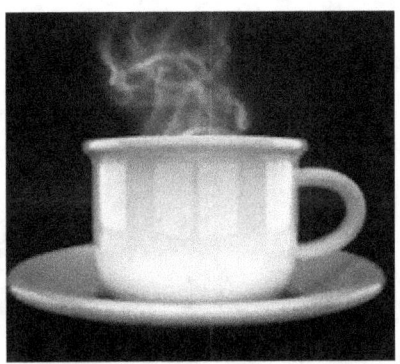

Hot water is great for maintaining a healthy metabolism, which is what you want if you're trying to shed a few kilos. The best way to do this is to kick start your metabolism early in the morning with a glass of hot water and lemon. As an added bonus, hot water will help to break down the adipose tissue (aka body fat) in your body. Drinking hot water is an excellent natural remedy for colds, coughs and a sore throat. It dissolves phlegm and also helps to remove it from your respiratory tract. As such, it can provide relief from a sore throat. It also helps in clearing nasal congestion.

Drink around 1 litre hot water on an unfilled stomach. This will cleanse the body thoroughly.

25. Ginger

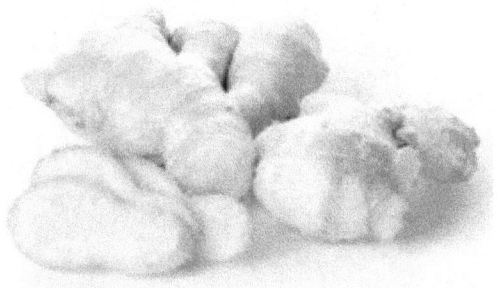

Ginger has a long history of use for relieving digestive problems such as nausea, loss of appetite, motion sickness and pain. The root or underground stem (rhizome) of the ginger plant can be consumed fresh, powdered, dried as a spice, in oil form or as juiceGinger is among the healthiest (and most delicious) spices on the planet. It is loaded with nutrients and bioactive compounds that have powerful benefits for your body and brain.

Steep water and add ginger to it. Then, add honey and pepper. Simmer it for 5 minutes. Honey helps in dissolving the fat while ginger and pepper will increase the metabolic rate.

26. Mint

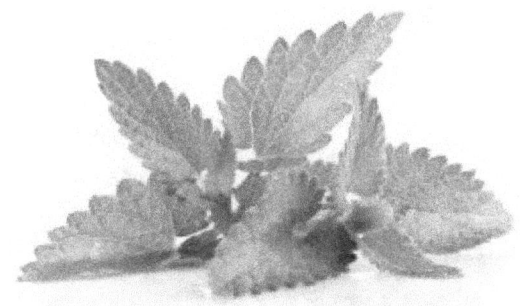

The health benefits of mint include the following: Digestion: Mint is a great appetizer or palate cleanser, and it promotes digestion. It also soothes stomachs in cases of indigestion or inflammation. When you feel sick to your stomach, drinking a cup of mint tea can give you relief. Fresh mint, including spearmint and peppermint, contains several key vitamins and minerals you need for good health, though they're not present in huge amounts. For example, fresh mint contains trace amounts of iron, a mineral you need to make red blood cells. Mint also has small amounts of fiber, vitamin A and potassium.

Add 1 tablespoon honey, a pinch of pepper, and some crushed mint leaves to a cup of hot water. Let it to steep for 5 minutes. Strain and drink the liquid to get a flat tummy. Mint soothes the abdomen while honey and pepper dissolves the fat and boosts the metabolism.

27. Curry Leaves

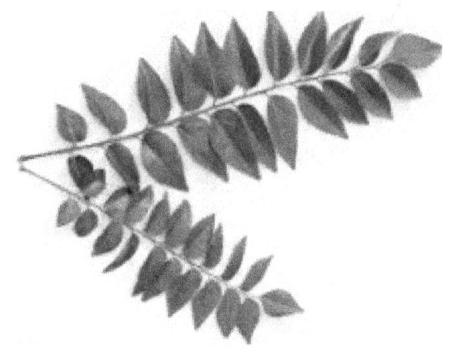

Curry leaves help in detoxification of the body, which automatically leads to less accumulation of fat on the tummy. Packed with carbohydrates, fiber, calcium, phosphorous, irons and vitamins like vitamin C, vitamin A, vitamin B, vitamin E, curry leaves help your heart function better, fights infections and can enliven your hair and skin with vitality.

28. Cardamom

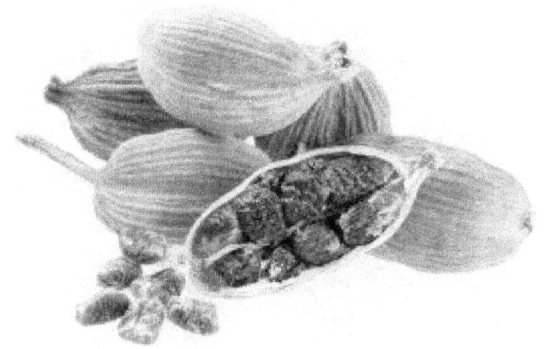

Cardamom is related to ginger and can be used in much the same way to counteract digestive problems. Use it to combat nausea, acidity, bloating, gas, heartburn, loss of appetite, constipation, and much more. This spice helps the body eliminate waste through the kidneys. Cardamom works as a great metabolism booster and an amazing detoxifying agent. Cardamom is also used for losing weight.

The health benefits of cardamom include gastrointestinal protection, cholesterol control, control of cancer, relief from cardiovascular issues, and the improvement of blood circulation in the body. It is useful for curing dental diseases and urinary tract infections such as cystitis, nephritis, and gonorrhea. Cardamom possesses aphrodisiac properties and is also used as a cure for impotency, erectile dysfunction, and premature ejaculation.

29. Almonds

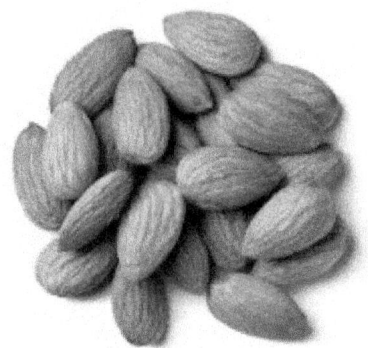

Almond is a rich source of vitamin E. Consumption of almonds makes you full for a long time, which means you eat less. Almonds are a source of vitamin E, copper, magnesium, and high-quality protein; they also contain high levels of healthy unsaturated fatty acids along with high levels of bioactive molecules (such as fiber, phytosterols, vitamins, other minerals, and antioxidants) which can help prevent cardiovascular heart diseases.

Cholesterol reduction is the most celebrated health benefit of almonds, but there are many other vital health benefits of almonds nutrition. Almonds are low in saturated fatty acids, rich in unsaturated fatty acids, and contain filling fiber, unique and protective phytosterol antioxidants as well as plant protein.

And don't fear the fat in almonds — almonds are actually beneficial when it comes to losing weight, despite their higher calorie content. One study even found that almonds consumed as snacks reduce hunger and desire to eat later in the day, and when dieters eat almonds daily they reduce their overall calorie intake.

30. Watermelon

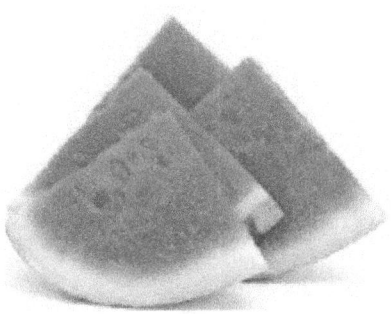

Watermelon contains 82% water, which helps your stomach not to crave for food. Watermelon is rich in vitamin C, which is beneficial for health. Phenolic compounds in watermelon—including flavonoids, carotenoids, and triterpenoids—make this fruit a choice for anti-inflammatory and antioxidant health benefits. If you had to pick a single nutrient from this anti-inflammatory and antioxidant category that has put watermelon on the map, that nutrient would be lycopene. Alongside of pink grapefruit and guava, watermelon is an unusually concentrated source of this carotenoid. Whereas most fruits get their reddish color from anthocyanin flavonoids, watermelon gets it reddish-pink shades primarily from lycopene. The lycopene content of watermelons increases along with ripening, so to get the best lycopene benefits from watermelon, make sure that your melon is optimally ripe.

31. Avocado

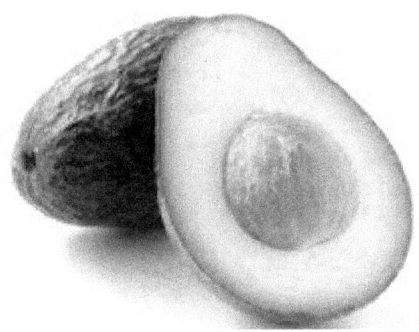

Avocado is a very useful fruit for burning the excess fat. Avocado is a rich source of fiber. It keeps the hunger at bay. The monounsaturated fatty acids in avocado help to reduce the belly fat. Avocados are very nutritious and contain a wide variety of nutrients, including 20 different vitamins and minerals. Avocados do not contain any cholesterol or <u>sodium</u>, and are low in <u>saturated fat</u>. I personally don't think that matters, but this is one of the reasons they are favored by many "old school" experts who still believe these things are inherently harmful.

32. Oats

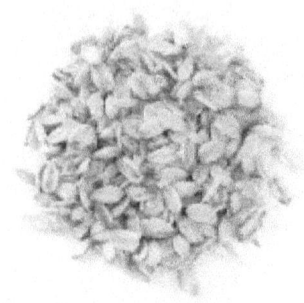

Oats are among the healthiest grains on earth. They're a gluten-free whole grain and a great source of important vitamins, minerals, fiber and antioxidants. Studies show that oats and oatmeal have many health benefits. These include weight loss, lower blood sugar levels and a reduced risk of heart disease.

Nutritional breakdown of oats. Dietary fiber - oats are rich in a specific type of fiber called beta-glucan. This particular type of fiber is known to help lower levels of bad cholesterol. One cup (81g) of dry oats contains 8.2 grams of fiber[1], the recommended daily intake of fiber is 25g for women and 38g for men. Have oats in breakfast. Usually, oats are filling, which means less hunger and less consumption of calories.

33. Apple

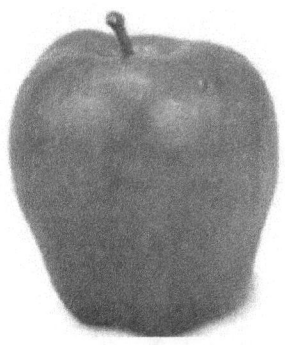

Eating apples regularly can help in fighting many diseases and it can also help in reducing the fat from your belly. Apple helps your stomach to feel full because it contains potassium and many vitamins. So, eat an apple in breakfast to get the desired tummy size. Apples are extremely rich in important antioxidants, flavanoids, and dietary fiber. The phytonutrients and antioxidants in apples may help reduce the risk of developing cancer, hypertension, diabetes, and heart disease. This article provides a nutritional profile of the fruit and its possible health benefits.

34. Juice of Cranberry

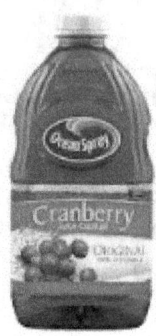

Drinking juice of cranberry can help in burning fat because it's rich in organic acid, which works as a digestive enzyme. Drink unsweetened cranberry juice daily for good results. The health benefits of cranberry juice include relief from urinary tract infection, respiratory disorders, kidney stones, cancer, and heart disease. It is also beneficial in preventing stomach disorders and diabetes, as well as gum diseases caused by dental plaque.

35. Peanut Butter

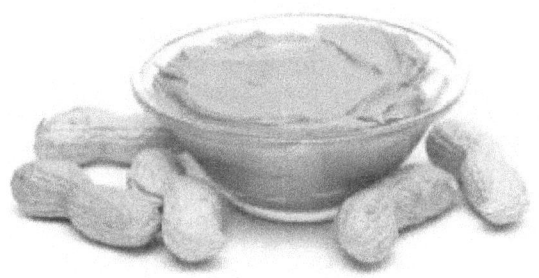

Peanut butter suppresses your appetite and boosts the metabolism. Peanut butter has niacin that avoids your tummy from bloating. Peanut butter has protein as well as potassium — which lowers the risk of high blood pressure, stroke and heart disease. It also contains fiber for your bowel health, healthy fats, magnesium to fortify your bones and muscles, Vitamin E and antioxidants

36. Eggs

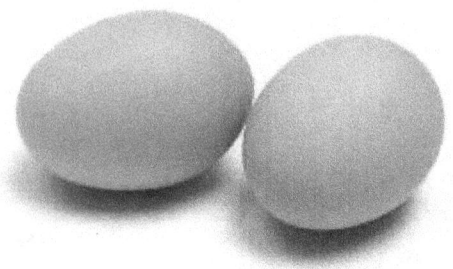

Egg is loaded with plenty of vitamins and contains calcium, zinc, iron, phosphorus, omega-3, etc. All these helps in burning the belly fat. So, grab an omelet in the morning for a flat belly. Eggs are a very good source of inexpensive, high quality protein. More than half the protein of an egg is found in the egg white along with vitamin B2 and lower amounts of fat and cholesterol than the yolk. The whites are rich sources of selenium, vitamin D, B6, B12 and minerals such as zinc, iron and copper.

37. Berries

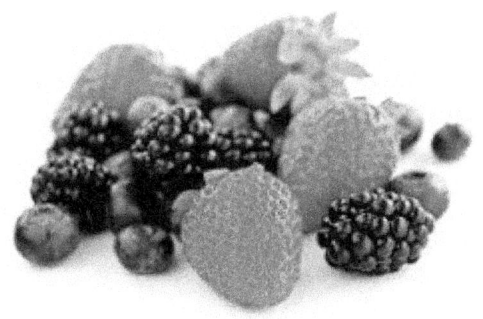

Strawberries, blackberries and raspberries contain plenty of fibers and are loaded with vitamins, which help to fight the cravings for food and sugary substances. This will slim down your belly. **Blueberries** are packed with antioxidants, called anthocyanins, that may help keep memory sharp as you age, and raspberries contain ellagic acid, a compound with anti-cancer properties. All **berries** are great sources of fiber, a nutrient important for a healthy digestive system.

38. Yogurt

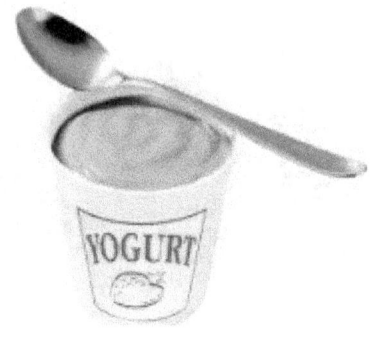

Though, yogurt can help in gaining more weight, but plain and Greek yogurt can help in cut down the excess fat from the belly. Eat only Greek and plain yogurt to reduce the fat. **yogurt** per day can provide protein, calcium, iodine, and potassium while helping you feel full for few calories. But maybe more importantly, yogurt provides healthy bacteria for the digestive tract which can affect the entire body. So yogurt eaters will get a dose of animal protein (about 9 grams per 6-ounce serving), plus several other nutrients found in dairy foods, like calcium, vitamin B-2, vitamin B-12, potassium, and magnesium.

39. Bottle Gourd Juice

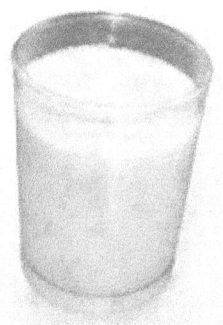

Juice of bottle gourd is very healthy. Drink a glass of bottle gourd juice for a flat and attractive tummy. Bottle gourd contains 96% of water and it also has dietary fiber, vitamin B, C, potassium and iron in very high quantity.

40. Parsley Juice

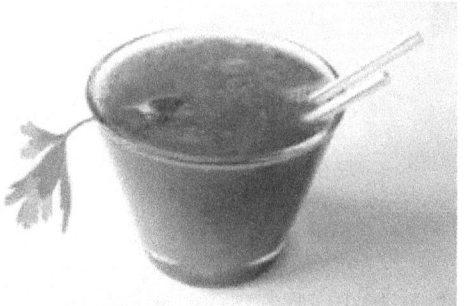

Parsley juice works as a detoxifier, which is filling as well as burns the calories. Parsley is an excellent herb for kidney and a great fat burner. Parsley is one of the best disease-fighting herbs and has been used as a natural medicine for centuries. The health benefits of drinking parsley juice range from bad breath treatment, cancer prevention, digestive and kidney support, anti-inflammatory effects and so much more. After just 2 weeks, your body will start to reap these amazing benefits!

Suffice to say, the properties of parsley are highly underrated, and need to get noticed. Parsley makes a great addition to salads, smoothies, and juices. I love making my fennel-parsley-ginger-lemon-apple juice – it tastes incredible and provides the body with a host of vitamins, minerals, and phytonutrients to help heal the body, protect it from harmful free radicals and enhance functioning of the heart.

41. Cayenne Pepper

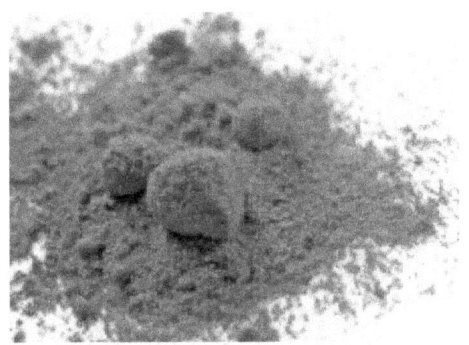

Cayenne pepper and ginger can help in clearing the lungs and flush out the fat from the body. Take cayenne pepper and ginger. Crush them together and have the mixture daily. Helps Digestion. One of the major cayenne pepper benefits is the positive effect it has on the digestive system. Relieves Migraine Pain, Prevents Blood Clots, Provides Detox Support, Relieves Joint and Nerve Pain, Supports Weight Loss, Works as Anti-Irritant, Boosts Metabolism. Cayenne is a well-known digestive aid. It stimulates the digestive tract, increasing the flow of enzyme production and gastric juices. This aids the body's ability to metabolize food (and toxins). Cayenne pepper is also helpful for relieving intestinal gas. It stimulates intestinal peristaltic motion, aiding in both assimilation and elimination.

42. Bananas

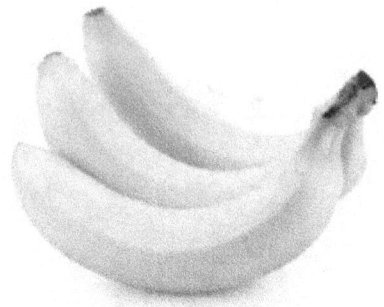

Like apples, bananas are also rich in potassium and contain multivitamins. They are filling and help you to resist the cravings for fast food. Moreover, banana boosts the metabolic rate, thereby melting the belly fat. Bananas are extremely healthy and delicious. They contain several essential nutrients, and have benefits for digestion, heart health and weight loss. Bananas are among the most popular fruits on earth. Bananas contain a fair amount of fiber, as well as several antioxidants.

43. Celery

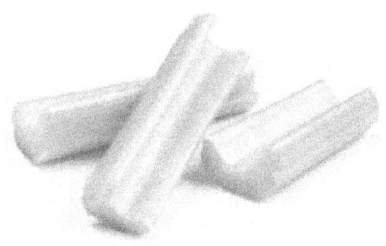

Celery also helps in reducing the fat from the belly and it contains only 8 calories. Drink celery juice or eat raw celery as a salad.

44. Grapefruit Juice

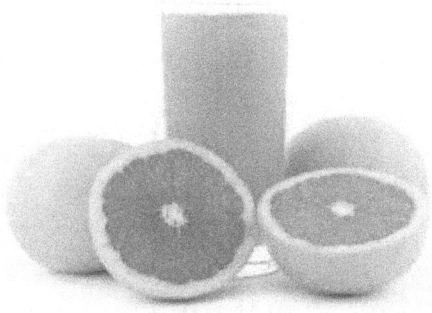

Grapefruit is being used for long time as part of body fat loss. It may help in weight loss either by reducing the hormone insulin causing reduction in weight. It could also be due to the fact it contains very low calories. When you take it before meals, you tend to eat less food later which can lead to weight loss.

45. Coconut Oil

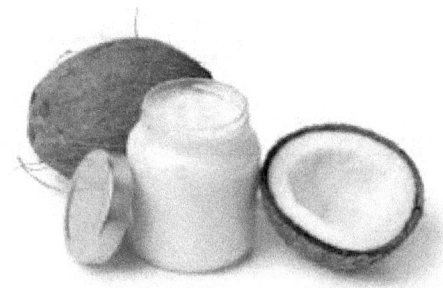

Coconut oil contains unique fats called Medium Chain Triglycerides (MCT) that help you burn calories more efficiently. MCT's are not stored away immediately as fat as these are not broken down in intestines. Instead these are sent to liver where MCTs are used as energy. Instead, they absorbed intact and sent right to the liver, where they are used as energy.

A study published by 2010 the International Journal of Food Sciences and Nutrition in 2010 suggested that coconut oil could not only help boost metabolism bust also assist in suppressing appetite.

The best option for maximum benefits, it is suggested that you use coconut oil as replacement oil. Two teaspoons of coconut oil is enough for daily consumption.

46. Lemon and Cayenne Pepper

It is a trick to lose weight fast though you would not appreciate the taste of the cayenne pepper. Add juice of one lemon and one teaspoon of cayenne pepper powder into one glass of water. You can add 2 tablespoons of maple syrup to add taste. Blend the mixer well and drink.

47. Honey and Yogurt

Yogurt contains probiotics which is very beneficial for digestive track and helps in maintaining a healthy balance of gut flora for optimized digestion.

Your body will be processing the food better when your digestive track is functioning smoothly.

You need one cup of plain yogurt and one tablespoon of honey. Mix both ingredients and eat at breakfast time.

48) Black Pepper and Lemon

Did you know that black pepper contains a naturally occurring chemical piperine that can interfere with the genes controlling the generation of fat cells. Piperine also reduces fat levels in the blood stream and enhances the absorption of nutrients from our foods. Lemon juice gives your digestion track a helping hand to break down foods. Add juice of one lemon in glass of fresh water. Sprinkle some freshly ground black pepper, mix it and drink once after a meal.

49. Cinnamon Tea

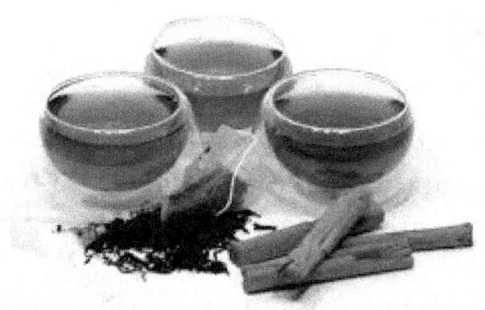

Cinnamon has shown to help manage blood sugar levels which has a direct impact on your weight as it affects how hungry and how energetic you are. You can prepare cinnamon tea by adding one teaspoon of ground cinnamon and one cinnamon stick to 8 ounces of boiling water. Let it steep for 15-20minutes and then strain. You can drink it 1-2 times daily.

50. Green Tea and Ginger

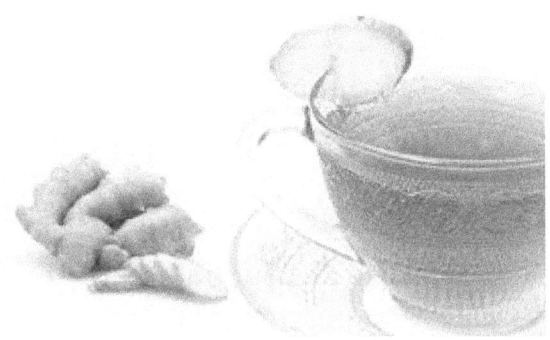

Green tea has caffeine that speeds up metabolism and some other body functions. Catechins in green tea can help lower the absorption of fats via the intestinal track. The ginger added to green tea will help improve digestion and add a little flavor.

In order to prepare green tea and ginger tea, steep half teaspoon ground ginger and one teaspoon of green tea in 8 ounces of boiling water for 4-5 minutes. For better results consume 1-2 cups of this tea empty stomach.

51. Rose Petal Water

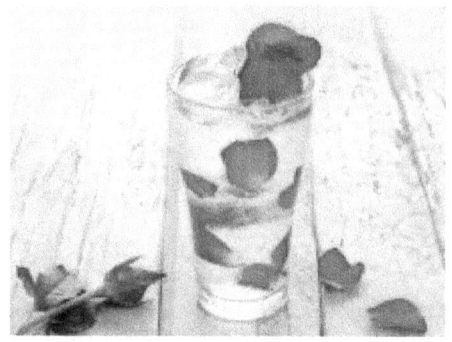

Rose petal water is diuretic in nature and thus encourages kidneys to put more sodium into your urine. The excessive salt (sodium) draws water from blood resulting in decreasing water weight. It will encourage you to drink more water to keep your body hydrated which is also beneficial in body fat loss.

You can add handful of dried rose petals to 1-2 cup of water (if possible use distilled water) and let it simmer for 15 minutes. Make sure that the pot which are using for preparing rose petal water has a lid that tightly fits on it. Drink half of cup of rose petal water empty stomach in the morning.

Effective Exercises to Lose Love Handles

Bicycling

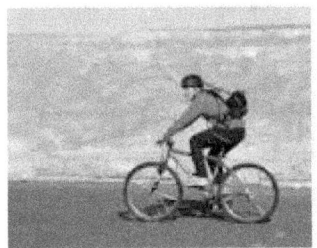

This is one of best known technique among the other home remedies for lose love handles fast. Cycling for a few kilometers every morning and evening will help the love handles tone down their rhetoric along with strengthening thigh muscles.

Jogging

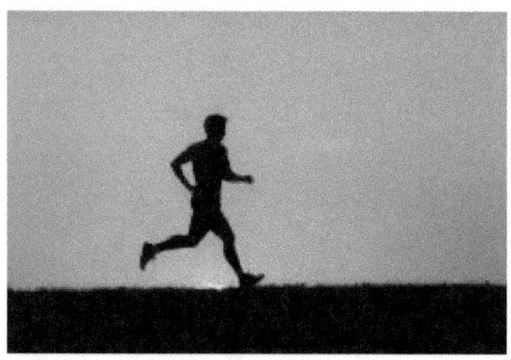

This is an easy way to bring intensity right to your belly and have the fat hanging around slim up. Go jogging early in the morning for best results and do it as long as you can sustain the pressure and intensity. Daily practicing provides guaranteed results but one can take it at four days a week if they can't afford the daily intensity.

Standard Crunch

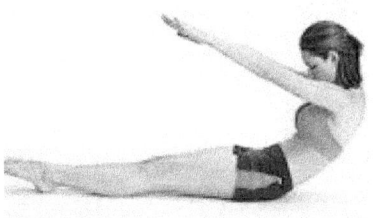

Crunches bring folding right to the waist line but you must be careful to take them slow lest you lose out on them. Start off with a minimal count then gradually increase every day for best results. Having them early morning and late evenings has proven effective for most persons.

Leg Flutters

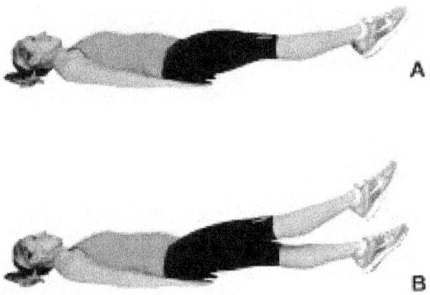

These are aimed at firming the abdominal muscles while strengthening the back. As the intensity and stretch catches up with the lower belly, the fat will be forced to melt away and leave behind the tough muscles without fat so you win the battle so easily. One has to lie on the stomach lifting their head then kick the limbs back and forth as long as you can.

Twisting Crunches

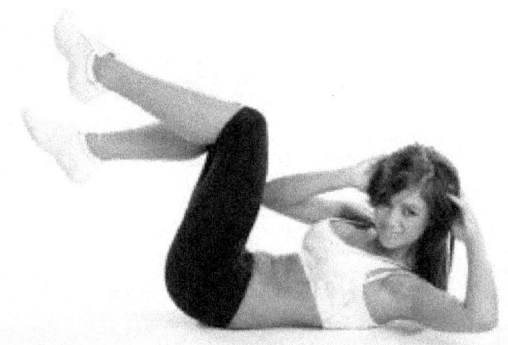

These crunches are much like the regular crunches except that a knee is raised and touched with an elbow of the opposite arm.

Standing Trunk Twists

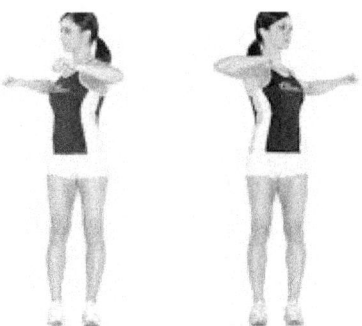

One needs to stand upright with a distance of about one foot separating the legs. Twist your trunks to the opposite side while occasionally punching in the air. Twenty five repetitions for each arm a day are a recommended set for optimal results.